BUILT TO LAST

THE ORIGINAL FITNESS GUIDE
FOR MIDDLE AGE

Start taking better care of yourself!

COLIN SOYER

No part of this publication may be reproduced, stored in a retrieval system, or transmitted in any form or by any means—electronic, photocopying, recording, or otherwise—without prior written permission, except in the case of brief excerpts in critical reviews and articles. For permission requests, contact the author at colinsoyer@verizon.net.

All rights reserved.

Copyright © 2021 Colin Soyer

ISBN: 9798732124538

The author disclaims responsibility for adverse effects or consequences from the misapplication or injudicious use of the information contained in this book. Mention of resources and associations does not imply an endorsement.

Table of Contents

Introduction 1

Welcome to Middle Age
(Background)

Chapter 1: The Middle of Your Life 5
Chapter 2: Your Life Today 9
Chapter 3: The Older Athlete 13
Chapter 4: The Aging Body 17
Chapter 5: Isn't Any Exercise Good? 23
Chapter 6: Look and Feel Younger 35

You Don't Mess Around with Gym
(Gaining Muscle)

Chapter 7: Put the Work in Workout 43
Chapter 8: The Program 45
Chapter 9: The Importance of Correct Form 55

Chapter 10: Volume and Intensity....................59

Chapter 11: Stretching and Warming Up 67

Chapter 12: Scheduling......................................71

Chapter 13: Useful Tips 81

The Cardio Solution
(Losing Fat)

Chapter 14: Aerobic Exercise 89

Live and Let Diet
(Eat Right)

Chapter 15: Nutrition......................................101

The Rest Will Take Care of Itself
(Recover, Restore, Replenish)

Chapter 16: Sleep 115

You Look Mahvelous
(Appearance Counts)

Chapter 17: Appearance 123

The Best is Yet to Come
(Inspiration)

Chapter 18: Believe 129

Chapter 19: Achieve 133

Chapter 20: Expect... 137

Chapter 21: Observe 143

Recap

Chapter 22: Taking Care of Business 149

Chapter 23: Never Give Up... 153

Chapter 24: Final Thoughts... 155

Acknowledgements 157

Introduction

You're not a kid anymore but you're not ready to hang it up either.

You're not a professional athlete but you're still active and occasionally athletic.

You know you should be doing something as you get older but you're not exactly sure what or how.

Think about it. What are you really after?

- Feeling better
- Looking younger
- Living longer

It's time to transform yourself.

We're not talking about just getting "fit" or finishing a race or any other competition with others or yourself.

This is about what you need to do individually to reverse the gradual wasting away that comes with age.

It runs counter to the natural progression of getting older, but it works.

Does it ever!

Welcome to Middle Age

(Background)

Chapter 1

The Middle of Your Life

*Forty is the old age of youth,
fifty is the youth of old age.*
— Victor Hugo (1802-1885)
French poet, dramatist and novelist

Yes, the middle.

Why am I saying this? Does it mean that if you're 50 you're going to live to be 100?

Maybe, but that's not what I'm talking about.

When you think of middle age you probably imagine adults in their 40s or 50s, give or take a few years at either end.

It could start in your late 30s and end somewhere in your early 60s.

There is plenty of variation depending on who you're talking about, but for most the average range is from 40 to 60.

I looked in dictionary.com for a definition of middle age. I came up with "the period between early adulthood and old age, usually considered as the years from about 45 to 65." Pretty standard.

Then I looked in thesaurus.com for synonyms for middle age. Not a lot there. There is virtually nothing, no other way to describe this period in life.

Almost like it doesn't exist or it's of no significance. There are plenty of words to describe youth and old age but nothing for the middle. How overlooked is that?

Is it taken for granted or considered so average and ordinary that nothing special is used to describe it? The only other synonyms are "midlife" and "the wrong side of forty."

Wrong side of forty?

Just the fact that there are so few synonyms for middle age tells me that this is a very neglected concept. Why is so little attention paid to midlife, especially as it relates to fitness and physical well-being?

I believe that this is underserved precisely because of where it lies.

In other words, you are either youthful enough to engage in vigorous physical activity or you are so advanced in age and feeble that you need to curtail your efforts and lower your expectations of results.

What is the ideal approach for someone in the middle? What works with this particular level of recovery ability and time constraint?

Many younger adults are well on their way to becoming physical wrecks, or are there already. Maybe a third of younger adults actually exercise with any regularity (and this is being generous). Out of that group, maybe half of them are actually achieving any significant results.

This means that over 80% of the younger adult population is aging poorly. And this is the group between 18 and 35! Imagine the numbers for typical people over 35.

Before we physically become adults, somewhere around age 18, our bodies are growing naturally and progressively. Soon after, growth slows and eventually deterioration begins unless active effort is made to counter this trend.

According to data compiled by the Social Security Administration a man reaching age 65 today can expect to live until age 84 while a woman turning 65 today can expect to live until 86 (https://www.ssa.gov/OACT/population/longevity.html).

And those are just averages. About one out of every four 65-year-olds today will live past age 90, and one out of 10 will live past age 95.

In addition, an ever increasing focus on health combined with advances in science and medicine probably means that these figures will continue to climb indefinitely.

If you think about when your life, as you know it today, really began it was most likely around the time you turned 25. Chances are this is close to when you got your first "real job" and moved out on your own. Maybe you were married, maybe not, but it was when you started to establish some level of independence.

Based on the Social Security numbers it's probably safe to say that if you made it this far you can expect to live until at least 85 and quite possibly a lot longer than that.

So if you consider the years from 25 to 85, then the real mid-point of your life is at age 55.

In other words, at 55 you still have half of your life left to live. Do you really want to spend all that time worrying and complaining about your body falling apart?

Our goal is to get the body to continue to grow and rejuvenate itself. Before and after middle age may require different approaches, but we are going to be looking at what works for the majority in the 40-60 age group.

Chapter 2

Your Life Today

A person is always startled when he hears himself called old for the first time.
— Oliver Wendell Holmes (1809-1894)
American author and poet

Ask yourself a couple of questions:

- Why is it so important to assess your physical condition at this point in your life?
- What is it that motivates you now to improve the size, shape and development of your body?

As you get into your thirties and beyond, look back and think about how you approached your life.

Still a Kid (under 18)

Sports, athletics, you did it all without a second thought.

You wouldn't have listened to anything we said anyway.

Young Adult (18-25)

You were at the peak of your athletic potential.

If you were serious about your physical condition this is where you would have done it.

Finding Your Place in the World (25-35)

Career, family and thinking about the future were most important.

Diet and exercise start to take a back seat.

Getting Ahead (35-45)

Nothing else matters.

Settling In (to career or occupation and getting compensated for it, 45-55)

Expenses are up and demands on your time are incessant.

Working Hard (55-65)

And starting to think about old age.

Retirement [maybe] (65-80)

Health determines the quality of your life.

80 and Beyond: Congratulations!

Hopefully enjoying the days you have left.

In middle age, it may be obvious, but it is critical to recognize that at this point in your life you are basically leading a sedentary existence.

Whether desk-bound, standing or supervising others, in most cases little is required in the way of manual physical effort and certainly not for prolonged periods.

Your level of activity is just not what it used to be.

Chapter 3

The Older Athlete

> *I will never be an old man. To me, old age is always 15 years older than I am.*
> — Bernard M. Baruch (1870-1965)
> American financier

At some point in your life your body stops growing. The natural growth cycle that occurs during childhood and into adolescence eventually ends.

And guess what happens next?

There may be a period of leveling off but ultimately, if left to its own, your body will begin to deteriorate.

Slowly at first, but over time the wear and tear will accumulate and the unattended body left to its natural course will begin breaking down.

A body that is trained to grow will not experience this to the same degree. Your body can continue to grow for years and even decades after the normal growth cycle has ended.

In addition, your body can also begin to grow again after years of stagnation or deterioration, if properly encouraged.

In other words, the right exercise, recovery and nutrition approach will trigger your body to grow long after it would have normally stopped.

In doing so you are directly opposing the effects of aging which contribute to the eventual wasting away of physical health.

Loss of Muscle

Why is muscle mass so critical to your health and wellness?

Muscle is living, dynamic, demanding tissue.

It forces your body to meet its requirements. It revitalizes and invigorates by pushing your circulation and respiration to give it what it needs.

You're either growing or shrinking. If you think that you are maintaining your body then you're probably in decline.

Losing a little fat does not change the inevitable loss of muscle.

In the next chapter, we will explore the condition that is associated with the loss of muscle due to aging.

It's not a disease or even a symptom of something else but it's real and observable. It's hard to say what's normal for people but the tendency to lose muscle mass as you get older is no joke.

Everyone knows that high level professional athletes start to experience a drop off in performance even around age 30, and even many of them are actually starting to lose muscle tissue.

The good news is that muscle can and will be added in response to the right kind of resistance exercise.

Age related loss of muscle strength and mass is not inevitable and can actually be reversed in middle age.

Growing Again

Basically, even after childhood, you'll be growing again. You always hear "I stopped growing at 18" or the old joke "I stopped growing taller and now I'm just growing wider" (ha ha).

But you will be growing again.

How about a bigger shoe size (no fat on the feet)? Or a bigger shirt that's looser in the waist? Wearing fitted suits that still need to be taken in around the middle?

You are youthful if you're growing and you're aging if you're not, plain and simple. You're either growing or shrinking.

There is no leveling off, that's a pretty small target.

You grow and grow until you stop at some point and then the reverse begins. The body will continue to grow if it needs to because of the demands on it.

This idea may not be the Fountain of Youth but it challenges the physical deterioration of age.

Building the body while it matures will neutralize aging.

Call it the Fountain of Middle Age. It's really not that hard.

You just have to do it right.

Chapter 4

The Aging Body

> *This morning when I put on my underwear I could hear the Fruit-of-the-Loom guys laughing at me.*
> — Rodney Dangerfield (1921-2004)
> American comedian

Adults in their 40s and 50s tend to laugh it off when the conversation turns to getting older. Someone makes a crack about how you're putting on weight or looking the worse for wear (or whatever), then you make a joke or two and change the subject like it's nothing.

But you can see it, maybe in the eyes or the body position.

The anxiety, the concern, the reality.

You're getting older and your body is breaking down and you're just not sure what to do about it.

Muscle Loss as You Age

One of the most significant ways in which aging changes your body is in the progressive loss of muscle mass.

The term used to describe muscle loss as you age is ***sarcopenia***. After the age of 50 or so you can experience up to 1% of your muscle mass wasting away each year.

Sarcopenia is not a disease or a condition and there is no consensus on what is normal for the average adult. However, it is reasonably agreed that being less active is a major cause of this muscle loss.

You find yourself gaining weight or having more trouble losing weight even if you're eating less than ever before. You're burning fewer calories and you're not doing anything differently.

Muscle burns more calories than fat so you won't use up as many calories as when you were younger.

Your body has begun to alter its composition to less muscle and more fat.

Fat belly is a symptom, not the problem. Spot reduction does not exist. The body deposits fat where it is genetically predisposed to accumulate.

Sarcopenia is getting a lot of attention in research and clinical practice. Why wouldn't it with the huge numbers of middle agers seen in the population?

There's not much agreement on how to handle this but the importance of exercise is always at the top of the list. But when it comes to specifics there is little consistency or consensus.

Fortunately, we know better.

Slower Metabolism - Longer Recovery

Along with the loss of muscle mass that comes with aging is the slowing down of your metabolism. And as if that wasn't enough, a slower metabolism usually means some loss or reduction in recovery ability.

Recovery time just takes longer as the metabolism slows.

Injuries take longer to heal and the body needs more time to recover from various stresses including the after effects of exercise, specifically resistance work.

Muscles (the ones that move your limbs and other body parts, i.e. skeletal muscles) use up by far the most energy in your body. As muscle mass decreases as you age so do your energy requirements decrease and the metabolic rate slows down accordingly.

You are now burning fewer calories than before, expending less energy.

Even when you are physically active you are burning fewer calories due to having less muscle mass. This is why your metabolism slows progressively, maybe a percent or two every decade even before reaching middle age.

Your approach to exercise needs to account for this.

Scheduling and cycling as well as volume, intensity and rest time all need to be managed and balanced very specifically for the middle aged trainee.

Too much or too little and the body will not respond by growing.

You may lose some weight or see some improvement in muscle tone but the real benefits of triggering lean physical growth and countering the effects of aging will not be optimized. Some things work better than others.

Age Management

There are areas of medical research and practice that seek to improve the condition of the aging body.

Age Management is the term applied to having concern with the quality and health of the individual in later years (https://www.cnn.com/2007/HEALTH/04/06/chasing.antiaging.med/index.html).

This is a substantial global industry especially when factoring in the sale of anti-aging products such as supplements, skin care cosmetics, hormone therapies and the like.

The age management industry relies heavily on medical doctors writing prescriptions for growth hormone and testosterone. The argument is that the body produces less of these hormones as it ages and that replacing them will keep the body in better shape.

A good deal of this business comes down to making a medical diagnosis of a hormone deficiency, i.e. low levels of testosterone or human growth hormone. This authorizes doctors to write a prescription to counter declining hormones in the body.

Of course there can be various side effects as well as a shutting down of the body's own ability to produce hormones. There are numerous detractors who claim that these side effects and potential risks outweigh the benefits but there are plenty of patients who swear by the treatments.

To a middle aged adult this may sound like a real solution to an inevitable problem that one encounters later on in life. However the practices seen in age management have yet to be conclusively determined as safe and effective.

Clearly there is something going on here.

But one thing is for sure, there is no denying that intense health consciousness and current demographic trends are driving a lot of attention to this field and creating a lot of interest.

Chapter 5

Isn't Any Exercise Good?

> *Be careful about reading health books.*
> *You may die of a misprint.*
> — Mark Twain (1835-1910)
> American humorist, writer, and lecturer

There are tons of books about exercise out there. Every conceivable variation has more selections to choose from than you could possibly ever get through.

And there are plenty that target older adults with specialized programs that are appropriate for those that have gotten on in years.

But as I mentioned earlier, all of these assume that you are either youthful enough to engage in vigorous physical activity or you are so advanced in age and feeble that you need to curtail your efforts and lower your expectations of results.

Here we focus on the ideal approach for someone in the middle, specifically what works with your midlife recovery ability and time constraints.

This program has been designed expressly for middle aged adults that are serious about their health and fitness.

It's not for kids or retirees that have hours to spend wandering around the gym socializing and catching up on the latest gossip.

It's not for anyone who's looking to "get into shape" to get the spouse off their back or to impress a coworker.

Also this is not the usual exercise manual that assumes you grasp nothing about weight training or fitness and then just goes on about how the enclosed instruction has everything you need to know.

This is for people that recognize the value of a well-built healthy body, have made the effort at some point in their lives, are looking for realistic guidance and are now ready to take the necessary steps to get where they aspire to be.

Beyond Fit

So what does 'being fit' mean?

I think it has something to do with not being too fat, having some visible level of muscle (I could say 'muscle tone' but then we're right back to what does that mean), and a cardio-pulmonary system that won't cut out on you after you walk up a flight or two of stairs.

Fitness then is a moving target.

What would pass for 'fit' at age 45 is a lot different than what would fly at age 25.

Middle age fitness is not enough to keep you from aging poorly because the standard decreases as the years go by.

With this program we are going beyond fitness.

Certainly the main elements will be there (lean body with strong heart and lungs), but we are concentrating on building up the muscle mass to oppose the inevitable physical degeneration that comes with age.

Building Your Body

First and foremost, it's about the amount of work you do.

If you want to counter the effects of age and the deterioration of your body, (muscles, bones, nerves) then forget about things like intensity, duration, cycling of routines, pyramids, circuits, advanced techniques, variety, etc.

High intensity exercise will certainly increase your heart and lung capacity. That's great if you live on the top floor of a 5 story walk up apartment house.

Building your body requires a different approach, and it involves work.

You build your body by doing an adequate amount of work to trigger the growth response.

There must be enough volume of effort applied with the proper form to get this outcome. The idea is to exercise more effectively and get real results.

This means your approach is a little bit longer, a little less intense and with a good deal more work.

Work equals more sets and reps, done progressively and with reasonably strict form.

The goal is to create a compounding or cumulative effect. In other words, continue to build on what you've already attained.

Muscular Development

Athletes who specialize in developing their musculature for competitive display or simply for health or fitness reasons are called bodybuilders.

Isn't Any Exercise Good?

The basic approach used by bodybuilders to get bigger muscles while keeping body fat at lower levels applies different elements of these three main features:

1. Resistance training involving some form of weight lifting
2. Attention to nutrition with an increase in protein consumption
3. Rest and recovery including extra sleep

Weight training breaks down muscle fibers and the subsequent repair of the muscle results in its growth (or hypertrophy). The size of the muscle increase depends on the type of weight training being used.

The main difference is that lifting for higher repetitions (the standard bodybuilding range is 8 - 12) increases the volume of the muscle cell while lower repetitions build up the muscle fibers that account for the muscle's strength.

All of this development demands a greater focus on the diet to ensure that there are adequate calories available to build muscle with and to provide energy for the training requirements.

Protein is consumed in quantities based on body weight, often going as high as 1 gram per pound or even more. Carbohydrates are thought of as fuel to provide energy for the body to respond to the demands being placed on it.

Carbs also promote the secretion of insulin which brings amino acids into the cells and encourages protein synthesis.

Muscle actually grows when the body is resting, not when muscles are being worked in the gym. Sleep provides the opportunity for recuperation and further development and it is critical to maintain appropriate habits and allow enough time for recovery to take place.

Hypertrophy

So we know that the whole point of this is to get the muscles to grow. But how does this actually happen? What goes on in the body that makes the muscle increase in size and strength?

A muscle grows in response to the demand placed on it. It adapts to the stimulus of weight training by increasing the volume of the muscle cell, either the dimensions of the contractile muscle fiber or the material within the cell.

The generally accepted thinking is that lower reps increase the size, and maybe the number, of muscle fibers and higher reps increase the mass of the muscle cell itself.

This response by the muscle allows it to become more effective at energy consumption. Most of the energy of the body is used by the muscular system and greater demands on the muscle cause it to adapt to become better prepared for the increased requirement.

Isn't Any Exercise Good?

The muscle cell's internal energy is in the form of ATP (Adenosine TriPhosphate). ATP is the molecule that carries energy to where it is needed in the cell. When ATP breaks down it releases energy that is used in the metabolic process.

This energy is used up very quickly when the muscle starts to contract.

Once the ATP is exhausted the muscle turns to its own glycogen (carbohydrate storage) supply for energy to continue contracting. In response to persistent higher demand the muscle will build up its glycogen storage.

It is this increase in glycogen reserves within the sarcoplasm of the muscle cell itself that accounts for a good deal of the size increase experienced when weight training in higher volume.

This process of growth and adaptation drives the body to renew itself. The increased energy demands trigger the body into a response of regeneration and revitalization.

Training Styles

We use different terms, like strength training, to describe the weight lifting part of the exercise program. But this isn't completely accurate.

Strength training, i.e. training to get stronger, is a different approach than our plan of action. True strength training is concerned only with how much weight you can move with proper form, not its effect on the skeletal muscles or overall health of the body.

Generally speaking you would use lower reps and longer rest times. A large part of building strength also comes from increased efficiency and better recruitment of the nervous system. These things are important but are not the primary focus of what we're doing.

The term weightlifting is also problematic. This is used to describe Olympic events as well as applied as a generic term for barbell and dumbbell work.

Then there is bodybuilding. This word implies many things beyond the resistance exercises. It includes diet, rest, competitions and all the other lifestyle elements that go along with it. So bodybuilding is not really just a style or program for lifting weights.

What we do could also be considered a version of volume training where the focus is on the amount of sets and reps done. Of course this is pretty simplistic and there's much more to it than just sets and reps, but it provides a good understanding as opposed to something like High Intensity Training or more eclectic methods such as CrossFit.

So let's call our style of weight training *Muscle Building* just to contrast that part of the program from the cardio. *Muscle Building* is the first component of the Built to Last method and it is essential to have a clear understanding of it right from the start. Focusing on the amount of work done in the gym is critical and it's about more than just strength.

In this program it's really about growth and what keeps the middle aged body from aging. There are plenty of other ways to approach fitness if your goals are different and if your interests go beyond looking younger, feeling better and living longer.

Fitness Lemmings

Muscle Building is not like jogging every day for 30 minutes. Or taking a group exercise class in your local gym.

Anyone can make you sweaty and exhausted. Run up and down a flight of stairs for awhile and find out how easy it is to get tired and worn out.

Is your exercise a means to an end or the goal itself? I read an email from a blogger discussing his pushups routine and how he tried to do more pushups each time. He then discussed his inconsistent form and realization that he could do more pushups if he did them faster. Obviously his goal is to increase the number of pushups he can do before muscular failure.

Is this you? Are you doing exercise for the sake of exercise? Or is the exercise a tool to use for a greater benefit. In this case a pushup is primarily a chest exercise and can effectively be used to contribute to building a bigger, stronger upper body and possibly even a greater systemic effect if performed properly. It would also be considered just a small part of a much larger overall routine designed to work the entire body.

Or are you just doing pushups?

Are you going to the gym pretty regularly now? What's really changed? Working up a sweat, getting a little sore, getting out of breath. Maybe your biceps got a bit bigger and your waist got a little smaller.

What do you expect to accomplish, or better still, what have you accomplished? Another rep on the push press or shaved 5 seconds off doing 20 burpees?

You want to be able to wear your accomplishments every day. You will see the progress in the mirror, carry yourself better and feel the confidence from knowing that you are improving yourself, and it shows.

Another pushup anyone? You can do better.

In Middle Age It's Not About Performance

It's about increasing muscle and decreasing fat. In other words, building up your body.

This is not about reducing or just losing weight. It's about expanding and developing, not shrinking down.

Isn't Any Exercise Good?

More lean muscle means a healthier, more youthful body.

You're not just training for strength (i.e. see how much you can lift) or for performance in some other activity (e.g. be a better tennis player).

Here are your exercise priorities for slowing down the aging process:

1. Gain muscle
2. Lose fat
3. Strengthen heart and lungs

In that order.

This is the precise, particular approach for middle agers. The goal is not to be the biggest, leanest or strongest but to be very advanced in all three areas.

You must put the time in and you must adopt the basic principles.

Chapter 6

Look and Feel Younger

> *Every person is responsible for his own looks after 40.*
>
> — Abraham Lincoln (1809-1865)
> 16th President of the United States

Greater muscle mass promotes a healthier, more youthful body. A physique is built by increasing lean muscle tissue, making you more injury and disease resistant.

As the body ages the amount of muscle will wither. Casual exercise to just stay lean and to work the heart and lungs will not counter the natural decline of muscle.

Remember the exercise priorities for slowing down the aging process:

- Only properly applied resistance exercise triggers the response that causes the muscle to grow.
- Correct nutrition makes available the nutrients that the body needs to increase muscle mass.
- Muscle growth and repair happens when the body rests, not when it's active.

Muscle Building works by prompting tissue regeneration:

- It renews the tissues that make up the body.
- It increases blood flow.
- It flushes wastes and toxins.
- It encourages new cell formation to replace older, less efficient cells.

This program is not for the typical sedentary overweight middle aged adult who is looking for a quick diet fix or an easy way to drop a few pounds.

Muscle Building is for the person who already recognizes the value of exercise and diet for a healthy and youthful life and is not getting the results they want from their current plan.

Muscle Gains and Fat Loss

Build the muscle and strip the fat. There is no contradiction for these two occurring at the same time if the approach is correct.

Muscle growth is stimulated by a particular form of exercise while fat loss is realized by another.

Gaining muscle is accomplished through proper resistance exercise done with the correct level of volume and in the right rep range.

The muscle must be able to take in adequate nutrition after being stressed. This involves consuming appropriate levels of protein to provide the amino acids that form the building blocks of additional muscle growth.

Losing fat is accomplished by burning calories from the stores of fat already in your body.

This requires a sufficient amount of time dedicated to burning off the readily available calories in your bloodstream and glycogen stores so that the activity will then proceed to utilize the calories stored as fat.

Usually this involves 20 minutes or more of sustained elevated heart rate activity to make inroads into the fat burning phase. Ideally doing the cardio after the resistance will take you into fat burning that much sooner since the resistance exercise has burned a lot of the readily available calories and the lower intensity cardio will burn fat stores that much more quickly.

It's Time to Take it to the Next Level

It's tough at the beginning. You don't know what you're doing. It's uncomfortable. It hurts. Everybody else is more advanced than you.

Don't give up, it gets better fast.

After a week or two you'll find yourself wanting to push it further. When you start seeing the changes in your body and your strength levels taking off you'll know you've arrived.

The phrase 'get in shape' implies almost anything will work. Improve the heart and lungs, shed a few pounds, lose an inch or two. If these are your goals then any regular exercise will do it.

Muscle Building is different and requires a specific protocol.

If you settle in with the masses I can guarantee one thing: the best you can hope for is mediocrity.

To get ahead and achieve don't follow the crowd.

Dawdle and fuss and life will pass you by. Before you know it the years have piled on, you look the worse for wear and your health has deteriorated.

Anyone will start getting stiff after two weeks of inactivity. Imagine how you must feel after two decades. Flexibility, strength and muscularity deteriorates and gets lost quickly.

You must keep up with your program consistently just to stay even. Dedication must be a priority if you want to actually make progress.

Get up and get out of bed. Don't stay up so late if you can't get going in the morning. You can accomplish more in one day than most people will in a month.

Don't be the person who roams around the gym trying every piece of equipment and spends more time on the cell phone reading emails or looking at last night's sports. This is like being the Jack of all Trades but the Master of None.

Skills are important and can get you far but nothing enables you to take charge of life like when you are in control of your own physical elements.

Building up your lean body mass, strengthening your bones and connective tissue and sharpening your nervous system response will go a long way towards not only slowing the degeneration of your body over time but reversing it and creating a superior material presence.

Yes it's hard and it's not intuitive. Yes there are specific methods and protocols that must be followed. But it's manageable and certainly achievable if the desire is there.

It's not like running, or the old Nike slogan 'Just Do It'. It has to be done properly using systems that have worked and were discovered by people that set out to do just that - build their bodies.

The 1960s and 70s bodybuilders mostly got it right. They found what worked through trial and error and sharing information as a community. They went wrong by taking performance enhancers and taking it to extremes. It got to the point where a typical person could no longer identify with them and eventually their methods were dismissed. The once non familiar curiosities had evolved into something else that only appealed to the hardcore fans.

Muscle Building is not about these extremes, but we are interested in the methods and lessons learned.

You Don't Mess Around with Gym
(Gaining Muscle)

Chapter 7

Put the Work in Workout

> *The greatest feeling you can get in a gym, or the most satisfying feeling you can get in the gym is... The Pump.*
>
> — Arnold Schwarzenegger,
> Pumping Iron (1977)

Put the work in workout.

Work is when something moves.

Not when struggling under a weight.

Not when resting between sets.

Not when shuffling around in a circuit.

You need to trigger a cumulative effect. The goal in the gym is to do an amount of work - not to increase effort. Work is simply the exertion of force to overcome resistance. You measure this by the amount of work sets that you do.

The key to success is in the title: "Work".

The difference between weightlifting and *Muscle Building* is the distinction between moving the weight and working the body. Most people don't put in enough time or use their time effectively. A body part must move a certain amount over a period of time, in other words you are doing targeted work. As the body adapts, the capacity to do work increases - this means that you can use more weight in the same amount of time.

If you are not making progress it's probably because you're not doing enough work. Or maybe you're not recovering from the work you are doing. Recovery is different from resting between sets. Most people wait too long and lose the cumulative effect that's so important.

Chapter 8

The Program

> *There are risks and costs to a program of action.
> But they are far less than the long-range risks
> and costs of comfortable inaction.*
>
> — John F. Kennedy (1917-1963)
> 35th President of the United States

The foundation of Built to Last training is *Muscle Building* and Cardio, specifically 20 sets of weight training immediately followed by 20 minutes of aerobic training. That's 20 work sets for 10-12 reps each. One, and only one, bodypart per training session. That's four or five different exercises for five or four sets each, respectively.

This corresponds into roughly a one hour total workout of resistance training and steady cardio exercise. In practice, a one hour exercise session translates to 5 minutes stretching, 5 minutes progressive warm up specific to the lifts that are to come, 30 minutes for actual strength training and 20 minutes on the treadmill (or similar).

The basic idea is to do one thing at a time. This means exercise one body part only and then let it rest. I know this may be a radical idea for many of you, but at this stage of your life it is essential to address recovery ability while still being able to make progress. We do this by working that one body part to the limit and then leaving it alone for a week.

When you work one body part at a time with higher volumes and lower rest time between sets you make greater inroads into the capacity of the muscle to do work. The increased growth response takes place during the longer rest and recovery phase.

Go to the gym. Put in the hour. Go home. Come back tomorrow. Repeat.

Don't jump right in on your first day and take on this kind of work load. You build up to where you will do 20 sets of resistance work for one body part at a time. Then this is followed immediately by the 20 minutes of Cardio.

Warm up on the first big, basic movement and you are then ready for all the sets to follow.

Start with the tougher compound moves, primarily barbell. Work these in the midrange. This is what builds muscle mass. Forget lock out and peak contraction.

Then include some isolation moves using dumbbells, machines and cables.

It looks something like this:

Leg Day

Barbell squat, hack squat, leg extension, leg curl

Start with a light set of squats for 15 reps or so.

Now start stretching (back, neck, shoulders, legs, hips, etc.) and then do another somewhat heavier set of squats for around 10 reps.

Add some more weight and begin your first work set.

Rest about 45 seconds and move on to the second work set.

Finish 5 work sets and move immediately to the hack squats. Go right to the work sets here since you've already warmed up the legs with the barbell squats.

Finish 5 work sets with about 40 seconds rest between them and proceed right away to the leg extension. Again, no additional warm up.

Complete 5 work sets with about 35 seconds rest.

Repeat the process with the leg curls and when you're done you will have polished off a productive 20 set training session in high volume style in about 40 minutes.

You don't have to worry about doing legs again for another week.

Time now for the 20 minutes of Cardio and you are done for the day.

Let me emphasize that you are using <u>work</u> sets. This is very different from pyramid sets (where you add a little weight to each set - these are generally used for increasing strength).

Notice the distinction between strength training and *Muscle Building*. Your routine is always built around the basics: Bench, Row, Press, Squat, Curl while maintaining that same ratio of weights to Cardio.

This is a full workout program for adults in their 40's and 50's. Whenever I read something that supposedly is geared towards the "older" athlete, whatever that means, it always says the same thing: warm up more, use lighter weight, harder to lose weight, don't recover as fast. Here is a comprehensive, A to Z system that fully details the approach best suited to the middle aged person as distinct from what is used by younger or older people.

Plus you know what you have to do ahead of time. No more walking around thinking "what am I going to do next?" No more wondering if you'll be doing more or less today. No more blowing off something and telling yourself you'll try to fit it in later.

Always keep in mind why you work out at this point in your life. Bottom line, it's primarily for health. You're not trying to make the team or simply impress the crowd (hopefully not). You don't have to kill yourself. Do the work in the right order with the proper form and get ready to change your life.

Five Steps for Muscle Building Success

1. Use heavy weight

    This is a relative statement. The weight used depends not only on your personal level of strength but on the rep range in which you are working. The weight should be heavy enough to just complete the last rep of the set but still have enough left over for all the reps in the next set. Don't go to failure but you should be coming pretty close on each set.

2. Use good form

    This means not only using proper bio mechanical form, but includes two essential points:

a) Maintain constant tension on the working muscles

b) Always keep the weight moving

Don't worry so much about full stretch and peak contraction. Focus on staying tight and moving smoothly through the turns at top and bottom. You are resting the muscle if you let the tension off or if the weight comes to a stop. The muscle should only be resting in between sets, not during.

3. Lots of sets and reps

   Think in terms of 20 sets per body part per week. Torso muscles are your chest, back and shoulders and peripheral body parts are the legs (quads and hamstrings) and arms (biceps and triceps). You should spend most of your time in the 8-12 (bodybuilding) rep range with occasional visits to the 5-8 (strength) range and 12-15 (endurance) range. Aim for four sets per exercise and five exercises per body part. You have to do the sets and reps to get the training effect and change your body composition. Stick with straight sets, one body part at a time. Leave the high intensity/low volume training for someone else.

4. Eat right

   Think about your protein requirements first. A good rule of thumb is to establish your protein intake per day per pound of bodyweight. Factor in your macro nutrient breakdown to complete the picture. There are plenty of free nutrition apps available that will help you calculate your calories and establish an eating plan. You can easily set up daily nutrition goals which target your calorie needs by activity level and whether you want to gain or lose weight. Arrange your macro-nutrients by setting the protein intake according to your target weight. Follow this by adjusting carbs and fat and you will have a realistic and workable plan in place.

5. Rest

   This can be the toughest part of the equation. Finding enough hours in the day to get adequate sleep can be harder than the actual workouts. Similar to sets and reps, think in terms of average hours of sleep per day per week. In other words, if you get six and a half hours of sleep from Monday through Friday and manage 10 hours Saturday and Sunday, then you can average seven and a half hours per day for the week. Also, go to bed earlier. Take a short nap whenever possible, even if just for a few minutes.

Precise Protocol

What you are reading here is a precise exercise protocol that has worked for decades.

It's not like jogging every day for 30 minutes.

If all you care about is setting a Personal Record or beating out the other guy then stick with CrossFit.

If you need variety it comes from mixing up the different exercises for each bodypart and keeping all other basic variables constant.

Always remember it's all about the numbers and doing the same amount of work in the same amount of time.

10-12 reps
4-5 sets
4-5 movements
1 body part per day
5 workouts per week

Equals 20 work sets per body part per week.

Or looking at it another way:

One hour per day
Ten minutes warm ups and stretch
Thirty minutes resistance
Twenty minutes aerobic

How do we get to working out five days per week?

Start out with a Full Body routine 3X per week. This can be Monday, Wednesday, Friday or Tuesday, Thursday,

The Program

Saturday. Keep it simple. Squat, Bench Press, Row, Press, Curls. Use 1 or 2 sets for each the first few times and then add sets until you can do 4 or 5 at the same weight in the 10 - 12 rep range. After a few weeks of this it's time to move on to the next level.

Next comes the Split routine. You are adding exercises and splitting your body parts over two days. This gets done twice per week, usually Monday, Tuesday - Thursday, Friday. For example, legs and arms are done on Mondays and Thursdays and chest, back and shoulders are done on Tuesdays and Fridays. Add 1 or 2 exercises per body part in addition to the basics from your full body routine and keep the total sets to around 20. Again, after a few weeks of this it's time to move on to the final level.

Now we are using the Single Bodypart routine. Each part of the body is exercised once per week over 5 days. For example, Monday legs, Tuesday chest, Wednesday back, Thursday shoulders, Friday arms. Here you will work up to 4 or 5 different movements for the same bodypart using 4 or 5 sets for each. Total sets should be around 20 when you are advanced and ready to take on this kind of volume. Plan on taking a month or two at manageable resistance levels before getting to this target number. Once you're there you have truly arrived and you can really concentrate on getting the work done.

Chapter 9

The Importance of Correct Form

> *That which does not kill us makes us stronger.*
> — Friedrich Nietzsche (1844-1900)
> German-Swiss philosopher

If the whole idea is to work the intended muscle rather than just lift the weight in front of you then it stands to reason that you must use the proper technique for the task at hand.

Using proper form helps to provide focus on the specific muscle being worked. Keeping the form tight means being reasonably strict and not using momentum or non-targeted muscles excessively to assist you.

In practice, this involves lowering the weight under control and lifting the weight smoothly and at a constant speed. A little bit of loosening of form is OK for the last rep or two of the last set of an exercise, but even this should be kept to a minimum.

Stricter form also lessens the possibility of injury by keeping the body properly balanced and aligned. Whenever your form loosens up you run the risk of muscles being out of position and then having to work in ways that they're not ready for.

The safest way to develop correct form is to use a weight that is light enough to get all your reps without too much struggle. By doing this you can progress consistently while avoiding injury and frustration.

Develop the habit of setting your body correctly at the start of every exercise. You should never be in a contorted, unnatural position. You should always have a balanced stance with good posture, back slightly arched, rib cage held high, head and neck neutral and looking forward.

For example, let's look at the bench press. You sit down on the end of the bench, lie down and grab the bar. You lift the bar up off the catches and lower it to your chest. Then you

The Importance of Correct Form

push the bar back up by extending your arms and lower it again until you get all your reps.

Sound pretty good so far?

Let's try it another way. You sit down on the end of the bench. Slowly lower yourself keeping your back tight until your shoulders make contact with the bench. Your arms reach for the bar as you position yourself so your chin lines up underneath it.

Now plant your feet squarely on the floor so that you just touch the bench with your butt and your back is slightly arched with your shoulders pressed down. Take a deep breath as your rib cage rises and the back of your head touches the upper part of the bench.

Make sure your grip is equal distance on either side of the bar and your forearms are straight and perpendicular to the floor. Lift the bar up and slightly forward, pausing briefly to get into the starting position.

Lower the bar slowly and under control and reverse direction as the bar just touches the high point of your chest while contracting your pectoral muscles to press it up. As it reaches the top you smoothly reverse direction to lower it back to your chest while keeping tension on all the working muscles.

The bar doesn't stop moving until all the reps are done and the set is over.

Which version do you think has the better form and gets the better results?

Tension & Movement

As described earlier, this means using proper form while maintaining persistent tightness on the working muscles and always keeping the weight moving.

The objective is constant tension with continuous movement.

Work in the mid-range. Don't worry about full extension or peak contraction. Big muscles work hardest in the mid-range. Accessory muscles are usually called in at the edges of the range of motion.

Concentrate on staying strict and advancing steadily through the turns. Resting will come between the sets. Once you ease off on the tension or pause during the set you are then resting the muscle.

This is the basic *Muscle Building* style of fitness that has never been well understood by the general public.

It's not high intensity or changing things up on a daily basis for variety. It's a steady, work-like approach. This is accomplished by using a moderate weight and higher volume of work. The goal is not to merely move the weight but to work the muscle.

Chapter 10

Volume and Intensity

> *My psychiatrist told me I'm going crazy.*
> *I told him, "If you don't mind, I'd like a second opinion."*
> *He said, "All right. You're ugly too!*
>
> — Rodney Dangerfield, 1921-2004,
> American comedian

Two critical elements of *Muscle Building* are volume and intensity.

Volume indicates the amount of sets and repetitions involved in the exercises being done for the body part in a single workout.

Intensity refers to the degree of force in the work being performed to move a weight that is heavy enough to just complete the target repetitions.

This basically means that you do a fixed amount of work in a set period of time - you're not trying to do more sets or reps in the same amount of time. You are doing the same amount (volume) of work at every session.

Progress comes from always lifting just heavy enough to finish the number of reps. Start as heavy as possible within the target rep range and complete all your work. You don't bang out reps at the end at a lighter weight just for the sake of completing a set.

As the body adapts, the capacity to do work increases - you can use more weight in the same amount of time (intensity). This continuing repetition is what transforms you.

The goal is to do an established volume of work along with advancement of intensity. This is very different than knocking yourself out trying to make every effort to complete a rep.

Progression

So how do we really make progress?

Work more in the gym.

Not harder, not longer, but more.

Volume and Intensity

Don't exercise longer hours but do more in a given amount of time. You need intensity, but that is not the difference.

Training to failure leads to burn-out. You never know how well you will do. This leads to the additional stress of trying to finish an unknown quantity.

I find that the more I push myself to the limit the greater the tendency to start skipping workouts or finding excuses not to go.

The solution is ...

Stay within the rep range. Always.

Reserve some extra time to work on pushing to new levels. Resistance increases gradually as your capacity to do work improves.

Stay within your range and focus on doing the work, not pushing yourself to do more each time. The long-term benefits and results come from this consistent, get-the-job-done approach and not from trying to set a new personal record each time.

And do not pyramid!

Pyramid sets are not work sets. They are basically a way to warm up to a heavy set or two. It doesn't work for *Muscle Building* because you are doing too many reps at lighter weight and not enough at heavier weight.

Pyramid lifting is not your workout.

Don't add weight progressively just to do one or two sloppy sets at your top weight. Pyramid to warm up and then put your effort into your work sets. These you do with your working poundages, all you can handle while staying in your rep range.

Pyramids are for power lifters and ego strokers. Occasional strength work is good to push your working weights up, but this is a means to an end. Keep the word "work" in mind all the time, i.e. workout, work sets, etc.

Work-Work-Work

Here's an example of a pyramid for the bench press:

95 x 20
135 x 15
185 x 8
225 x 5 x 5

The *Muscle Building* way looks a little different (assuming the same level of strength):

135 x 8
185 x 5
205 x 12 x 11 x 10 x 10

The lighter sets happen during your stretching and warmup which are done together before the workout begins. You are only doing enough reps to prepare the body to do the heavier work sets.

There is little to be gained from the warmup other than that. Too many people do far too many pyramid sets and not enough work sets which reduces the volume to an ineffective amount.

It is absolutely critical to count reps. Get into the habit of utilizing a cadence of 3. Think of each count of three almost like a mini set. Focus on the feel of each rep without worrying so much about completing the set.

1,2,3 - 4,5,6 - 7,8,9 - 10,11,12

Try it and really pay attention to the cadence. You will find yourself getting into a crisp and efficient rhythm and soon enough it will become second nature.

Strength

Please let me make one thing perfectly clear:

You train for strength only to do your work sets better. The stronger you get the more weight you can use on your work sets.

The strength training is not the workout. It doesn't get the results that we're looking for. These are two different things with two different approaches.

It's fine to occasionally work on a dedicated strength program. Focus on one bodypart exclusively for pure strength and power.

For example, push your squat poundage by adding a little more weight each week. Don't worry about the number of reps. Just do 3-4 sets with increasing poundage from week to week for a month or so. The other leg exercises can stay in the 10-12 rep range or if you're feeling particularly good maybe push the weight in one or two other exercises. Maybe add some plates to the hack squat but keep the leg extensions and leg curls the same as usual.

The important thing is that the weight in the first big compound movement goes up over a period of time. Your body will let you know when you've had enough. Either the weight will plateau or your enthusiasm for this strength phase will wane.

Then its time to work on another body part or just go back to the standard routine (which works so well!) until your body lets you know its time to push the poundage in another body part.

Don't worry - you'll know when it's time. The exercise will call out to you. Time to get my bench press up!

Lifting in the low rep range will help to increase your strength. This does nothing for your body composition, i.e. losing weight or adding muscle. Strength training should only be used as a means to be more productive in your real work sets.

In other words you build your strength up so that you can now lift 185 for 12 in the squat when before you were using 135 for 12. To get to 185 for 12 you may need to spend several weeks lifting 225 for 5. The 225 for 5 does nothing for your fitness goals in and of itself, but when you go back to your 12 rep sets going heavier you are now adding muscle and burning fat like never before.

Strength is a tool to do more work. Strength lets you do more and better work. The problem most people have is that's all they do. They lift for strength.

Chapter 11

Stretching and Warming Up

All bodies are slow in growth but rapid in decay.

— Publius Cornelius Tacitus (55-117)
Roman historian

One of the first things you should do in the morning is stretch your spine. Nothing will age you faster or make you feel worse than a bad back. Start to become aware of the condition of your spine and begin to develop a sense of what's going on with your back.

Before you even warm up for your exercises you really need to get this done. Up, down, backward, forward, side to side and turning/twisting. Include the neck in all directions.

Just sleeping with your head propped up on a pillow or sitting at a desk leaning in to see a computer screen will cause your neck muscles to strain in different ways, often for prolonged periods of time.

This is not just about avoiding injury or trying to be more supple. A strong, well maintained spine will drive your overall health and vitality more than almost any aspect of your physical being. The back is the foundation from which your arms, legs and torso muscles all operate. A healthy spine lets the rest of your body get stronger, obviously improves your posture and reinforces your positive outlook on taking control of your life and actively managing the aging process.

Get in touch with your back, learn how to stretch your spine completely and enjoy the endless benefits that follow.

Clearly it's very important to warm up adequately before starting any serious exercise or other physical activity. The body needs to be prepared for what it's being asked to do both to avoid injury and to get the form right before it gets too demanding.

But there's another aspect to warming up that's often overlooked, and that's the mental side. There can be a reluctance or resistance to starting something that you know is going to be uncomfortable or require a great deal of effort. By starting easy and doing things that are not very demanding it becomes more acceptable to the mind and body.

Light stretching and weightlifting with easy poundages shouldn't be a problem regardless of your state of mind or level of fatigue. Once you get going it becomes easier to make incremental progress up to the point where you're going heavy in your work sets.

Where the mind goes the body follows.

Chapter 12

Scheduling

Remember, today is the tomorrow you worried about yesterday.

— Dale Carnegie (1888-1955)
American writer

Let me make this simple: if you don't schedule you will fail.

Be aware of the difference between weekdays and weekends. Schedule by day of the week, not some arbitrary cycle pattern.

Find the time of day during the week that allows you consistency.

Structure your exercise time accordingly whether it's first thing in the morning, right before bed in the evening, during lunch break, etc. You can be flexible on the weekend but schedule your time anyway and skip or reschedule only when necessary.

Schedule regular time for additional supportive tasks like prepping meals, packing clothes if you take them with you, naps (10-15 minutes when you really need it works wonders; obviously you need to be discrete if you are in a workplace or something similar), anything else that needs to be addressed ahead of time.

Only two significant things work against you during middle age: recovery ability and free time. Recovery must be managed by optimizing your training schedule and free time must be used in the most efficient manner possible.

The worst thing you can do is waste your time.

If there's anything sadder than an overweight, out of shape middle aged adult it's the one who actually makes the effort to go the gym and gets absolutely nowhere.

Pros and Cons

You must find that repeatable time during each and every day of the week.

Mornings

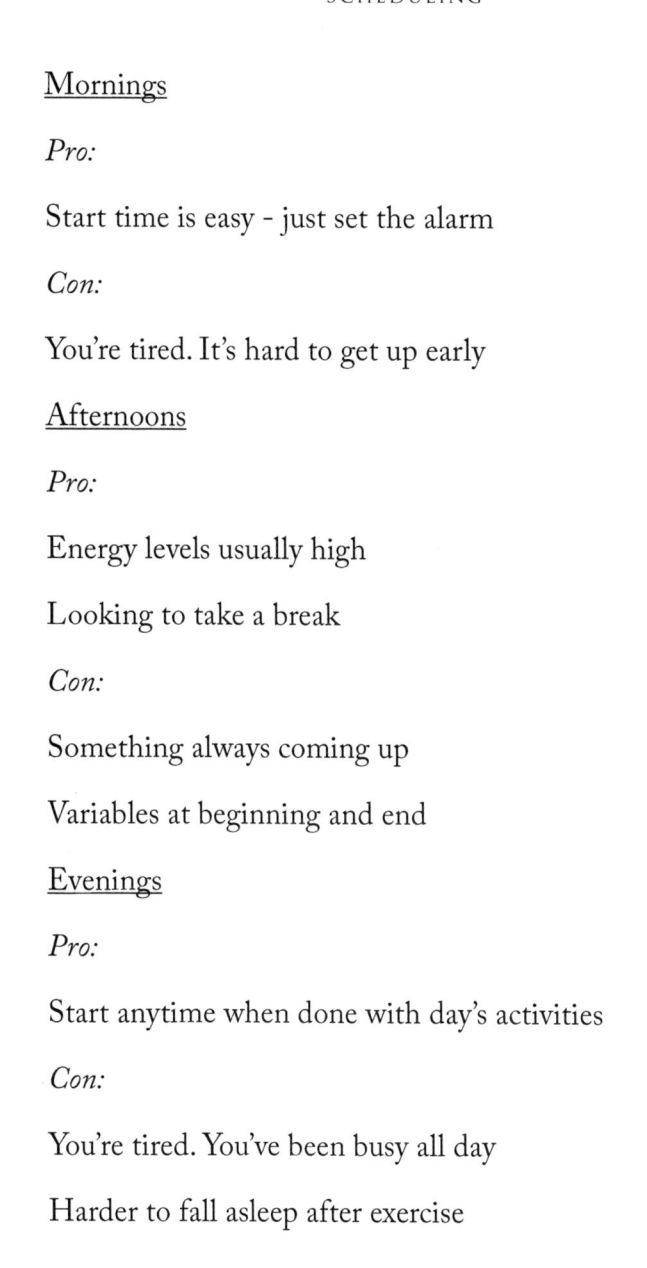

Pro:

Start time is easy - just set the alarm

Con:

You're tired. It's hard to get up early

Afternoons

Pro:

Energy levels usually high

Looking to take a break

Con:

Something always coming up

Variables at beginning and end

Evenings

Pro:

Start anytime when done with day's activities

Con:

You're tired. You've been busy all day

Harder to fall asleep after exercise

An Hour a Day

If you're really serious about making this work there is one simple solution:

Get up an hour earlier. That's all we ask.

- Go to bed an hour earlier
- Just get one hour less sleep
- Take a nap or two during the day
- Make up the lost hours on the weekend
- Or you can try some combination of the above

Three simple steps to getting started:

a. Set the alarm clock an hour earlier
b. Get out of bed when the alarm goes off
c. After that, the rest is easy

Allow time for your body to wake up in the morning. Find something productive to during this time.

An hour a day is all we ask.

Think of all the things you do that waste that much time. (iPhone anyone?)

You can do this!

The point is there's no excuse. It can be done.

You just have to want it and commit.

Mid Life Reality

Here is the reality of middle age.

You've been married for awhile now. Have a kid or two. You work a regular job, Monday to Friday, 9 to 5, weekends off. You might sit at a desk all day staring into a computer terminal or talking on a telephone without moving for hours at a time.

Remember when you used to get off from work and head right over to the gym for an afternoon workout? The gym bag was in the car or under your desk and you could leave and be there in minutes without having to stop home or telling anyone where you were going.

Over the years your responsibilities have increased. You never leave the job at the same time. Of course when you do leave it's time for dinner with the family. Most nights they wait for you to come home unless you're going to be really late at work. And you want to spend some time with the kids before they go to bed. Reserve some time with the spouse for those all-important discussions and the day is pretty much over.

The weekend comes and everything changes. You're going to get out of the house and hit the gym and make up for all the days and hours of inactivity. But you forgot about the errands, the kids' ball games, the home repairs, the yard work, and the relatives coming for a visit. Saturday and Sunday fly by and maybe you got in an hour of exercise, but it certainly didn't make up for what you missed during the week. Monday arrives and the cycle repeats itself all over again.

You lead a different life during the week and on the weekends. Five days on one schedule and two days on another. This particular fact is unlikely to change anytime soon and will be a part of you until you reach retirement age. The challenge is in finding the balance between family, work and your own personal goals.

Going to the gym regularly after work is out unless you are looking for your family to treat you like a stranger. Maybe you can make it once or twice a week at night without repercussion but will that be enough for you to get in the shape you know you're capable of? Get in an extra workout or two on the weekend and it looks like you may have a real program in place.

But how consistent is this going to be? Visiting the gym at the end of the day after the job and the family dinner when everyone wants a piece of you is not the easiest thing. Those good intentions for the Saturday or Sunday session have a way of getting pushed aside when other priorities appear. This hit or miss approach is typical of the middle aged adult's workout pattern and will only lead to frustration and failure if you can keep it up at all.

Every weekday the alarm clock goes off and you get out of bed. Head to the bathroom for a shower. Get dressed, maybe grab a cup of coffee and start the commute into work. This routine never varies. On the weekend, you probably turn the alarm off. Maybe you get up early, maybe you don't. You might get dressed right away or you might stay in the clothes you slept in.

The point is that the weekday routine is consistent and repeatable. It is automatic. You do the same things in the same order day in and day out. This is where your training belongs. By working out in the morning before the day begins, you have eliminated most of the distractions and excuses that can interfere with your training. What do you have to give up to make this happen?

The critical change is that you have to wake up earlier than you have been doing. Does this mean giving up hours of sleep? Not necessarily. Go to bed a little earlier in the evening and get out of the house a little quicker in the morning and you will have made up most of the time difference. Your family will certainly understand the need to get to bed earlier. Whether they recognize the importance of your fitness goals or not, don't you think the family would rather see you home in the evening than watch you racing out the door to go to the gym as soon as you get home from work. Going to sleep an hour or so earlier is a reasonable tradeoff if you spend most of the rest of the evening with the family. And think about how much you will be able to give your family when you have energy and a positive mindset.

The other piece of the equation is to be ready in the morning so that you can leave the house quickly. Have the gym bag packed with everything you need before you go to sleep. Hang your work clothes and bring them to the gym on the hanger. Shower at the gym after you work out. Your meals should be put together and waiting in the refrigerator. If you need that cup of coffee for the ride in, set up the coffeemaker the night before so you only need to flip the switch in the morning. Better still, use a coffee machine with a timer and have it brewed and waiting for you when you get up. Everything that goes with you should be prepared the night before and left where you can just grab it on your way out of the house.

Don't overlook the meal preparation. You should bring your food, don't buy it. A daily eating plan high enough in protein for the hard training middle aged adult cannot be maintained by trips to the deli or the cafeteria. Pack enough for three or four small meals and supplement with a quality protein powder and you won't miss the junk that you would normally buy. It also helps that you know exactly what you're eating when you prepare it yourself. Try to figure out from a nutritional standpoint what's in the typical deli sandwich and the advantages of packing your own meals will become very apparent.

The drive and determination comes from within. Managing the external forces can be as tough as or tougher than the program itself. By putting yourself on a consistent and repeatable plan of action, and with a little guidance from someone who has been there, your goals and all the associated benefits will well be within reach.

Chapter 13

Useful Tips

> *When I was fourteen, my father was so ignorant I could hardly stand to have him around. When I got to be twenty-one, I was astonished at how much he had learned in seven years.*
>
> — Mark Twain (1835-1910)
> American humorist, writer, and lecturer

Do not train to failure. Always save something for the next set.

Use working poundages in good form for 10-12 reps with managed (1 minute or less) rest time.

Start big and warm up slowly. Do your main compound move first and then move on to the smaller exercises. Stretch out in between warmup sets. This allows you to combine your stretching and warmup making it more productive for both and certainly more time efficient.

If you feel the need to look at your smartphone in between sets then you are resting too much. Focus! Prepare yourself for the next effort. Concentrate on what you're doing. When you get to Cardio your mind can wander or catch up on the news. Not between sets.

Rest only as long as you must to be able to complete the next set with the target number of reps and with good form. Shoot for 60 seconds rest in between sets. You may not be 100% fully recovered, but you should be able to hit your rep target on each set.

Reduce the rest time more with each successive exercise. These should be the smaller, less exhausting moves as you get to the later lifts. This approach will steadily increase the pace and the overall metabolic effect.

You can ease up on form a little as you move to later exercises but the big basic moves must be heavy, in good form, tight, and end just short of failure at the target rep number.

Intensity can be varied many different ways, e.g. the length of rest between sets will change intensity on the same exercise even when using the same weight.

Always apply continual refinement to find the optimal blend of effort and rest while staying in the *Muscle Building* rep range. Each set should be challenging while maintaining the least amount of rest needed to perform the next set properly.

Use the one body part per day method. The training effect comes from the cumulative work load. This is the main reason why circuit training doesn't get results. Circuit training is the worst. Too much time is spent resting one body part while you work another one.

Start pressing movements with full extension and lower just slightly enough to engage the muscle before beginning the set. This makes a surprisingly huge difference. Do not worry about full range of motion. Stay in the range that keeps the muscle engaged.

Relax the tension a little. Control, don't resist. Let the body find its own rhythm and let the movement find its natural groove (path). Don't resist the lowering weight or fight it. Just use enough effort to control it on the way down. You will get in a better rhythm, with less fatigue, and be able to conserve your strength for the actual lifting. The benefit of concentrating on the negative is dubious at best. Remember rhythm and groove.

Forget repping out, full extension, personal records and all the rest. Keep it tight, control the negative and keep the weight moving. Don't extend fully on the negative or you will lose the tightness.

Count by threes. Establish a rhythm. It's easier on you psychologically and the set will go more smoothly.

If you're not there mentally then start slow and don't think about it too much. You may get a great workout.

Keep it simple when you're first starting out so as to get the scheduling down. 20 minutes resistance training and 20 minutes aerobic three times a week. That's two hours to transform your life and take charge of your health. Carve out 40 minutes when you first get up or before you go to bed on three non-consecutive days. Tell yourself it's only 2 hours a week to change your life and before you know it you will own this forever.

If you're out of shape you can do almost anything physical on a fairly regular basis and initially your body will respond. These results may seem desirable compared to where you came from but nowhere near what you are capable of if proper methods are employed.

You need to own your training. To be entirely dependent on someone else to motivate you and steer you down the right path is simply a formula for failure. You have to make this a part of your life, same as you know you have to eat, go to work every day (or school), pay your bills on time and so on. It's not something you do for a period of time and then it ends.

Useful Tips

Whatever your goals are somewhere along the line you will go off track. Don't dwell on it. Pick yourself up and get going again. Everyone gets derailed at some point. The difference between achievers and everyone else is getting back on track and moving forward.

The Cardio Solution
(Losing Fat)

Chapter 14

Aerobic Exercise

> *Our fatigue is often caused not by work,
> but by worry, frustration and resentment.*
> — Dale Carnegie (1888-1955)
> American writer

Built to Last is not just about lifting weights. The other major fitness component we need to concern ourselves with is aerobic exercise (often called Cardio) which has distinct energy characteristics.

Cardio is simply continuous exercise done over a fairly long time interval at a moderate pace. A clear example would be jogging on a treadmill for awhile at a comfortable level.

Contrast this with walking on the treadmill (which would not be intense enough to be aerobic) or sprinting on the treadmill (which would be a much shorter length of time at a much higher level of intensity).

The biggest difference for our purpose is how energy is involved within the muscle. The time span and magnitude of muscle activity determines whether the exercise becomes aerobic or not.

When you start doing Cardio the first thing that happens is that muscle glycogen breaks down to produce glucose. Glucose is the main source of energy in the body and glycogen is the predominant form of storage for glucose.

As you continue your physical activity, the amount of glycogen in the muscle gets used up and the body needs to find another source of glucose. Energy then begins to get sourced from stored reserves of fat which release glucose to function as fuel. Continued exercise at roughly two-thirds of maximum heart rate will trigger the most fat burning.

It takes about 20 minutes to burn through your muscle glycogen. Why not use your weight lifting to do that? You're going to be burning it up anyway. Then when you hit Cardio after lifting you go right into fat burning. Twenty minutes of Cardio following your weight lifting means your body will be primed to burn more fat as you complete your workout.

Doing weight lifting, which mostly burns glycogen, before Cardio ideally positions you for optimum fat burning.

With Built to Last, Cardio is done for the purpose of bringing down body fat levels. We are not necessarily looking to lose weight or body mass. Our objective is always to increase muscle and decrease fat. By addressing these two things somewhat independently we can accomplish both at the same time.

However, there are some additional benefits that come from doing Cardio consistently:

- Your heart and lungs are invigorated leading to more efficient breathing and circulation.
- Red blood cells multiply resulting in better use of oxygen.
- Endurance improves as the body elevates the storage of energy in the muscles.
- Your recovery ability strengthens and your metabolism gets raised.

Cardio needs to be done regularly and with the required time component to achieve the desired outcome. Our program treats Cardio as an essential element to be performed at every workout, generally twenty minutes should do it. You don't undertake it separately as a stand-alone exercise but more as a continuation of the training routine after the lifting is done.

When done in this fashion the whole problem of "fitting it in" ceases to exist and it becomes automatic. Before you know it your body will be responding and doing it becomes almost effortless.

Types of Cardio

Almost any sustained activity at an adequate level of exertion while using your legs could be considered Cardio. Since our approach is to perform Cardio right after finishing a weight training resistance workout, it would probably be easier and more sustainable to find a suitable piece of equipment in the same gym.

However, this is one of those situations where sampling different options before settling on a favorite might go a long way towards keeping the motivation up and continuing with the program. You may want to mix it up, alternate indoor and outdoor, or just stick with the same thing every day.

The important thing is that your Cardio is done consistently and routinely. As log as it's the right kind of exercise and it's done properly it won't make too much difference which one you use.

In the Gym

Treadmill
Elliptical

Rower
Stationary Bike

Outside the Gym

Running
Jogging
Walking
Jump rope
Cycling

Running

A quick note about running.

One of the more common trends among adults who are looking to get back into shape after a long layoff is to lace up the old sneakers and hit the pavement. Running and jogging are excellent Cardio activities and many people participate, some regularly and some only occasionally.

While you may feel prepared by stretching out and waiting for a nice day to arrive, there are a few concerns that you should give some thought to ahead of time.

Stress on the joints:

Lifting your foot and bringing it back down over and over again will, at the very least, beat up your ankles and knees. If your body has not experienced this type of trauma in a while it won't take long for the pain to remind you and an injury is likely to follow.

Cardio-pulmonary limitations:

Your heart and lungs will be taxed very quickly to the point of discomfort, seriously hampering the duration of your effort. You may be slowing to a walk before any Cardio benefit is realized.

Muscle conditioning:

Even if you loosen up well, your legs and other muscles are being put in an extended state of tension that they haven't been called upon to do in some time. You may experience cramping or even injury before even realizing that this is happening.

If you really want to start running, or get back into it after a long while, the best way to approach it is to start slowly and increase the distance each time out. Start your run with a fairly brisk walk for 10 minutes or so. This gives your circulatory system a warm up and primes your joints and muscles for the more aggressive activity to follow. Break into a jog when you're ready and keep the pace steady until you finish. When you come out again the next time, in a day or two, start again with the walk and extend your running distance by a safe and manageable margin. Keep this up and pay attention to how your body feels afterward and you should be able to avoid most of the problems that

AEROBIC EXERCISE

would make you quit after only a couple of unproductive and agonizing sessions.

The Cardio Solution

So back to the title of this section.

Why do you need a solution for Cardio?

Because it's boring!

I used to hate doing Cardio until I figured it out. Now you can't get me off the machine. I'm actually disappointed when my session is over or I run out of time.

The trick is: *Do less more often.*

Make it easy to be repeatable. Same machine, same resistance, same motion, same effort. Do it the same way every time and you won't have to think about it.

No more "Oh no, it's Cardio day. What excuse can I come up with this time." Carve out your Cardio time at the end of each and every gym visit and you've taken all the pressure off for getting your Cardio work in.

This is way better than trying to get it all in over 2 or 3 sessions per week which you will come to hate. You have no idea how creative you can be when it comes to avoiding the dreaded lengthy Cardio session.

Most of these commercial exercise programs that get so popular are nothing more than versions of Cardio regardless of what they claim to accomplish. The expensive boutiques and at-home courses charge pretty high rates to do nothing more than elevate your heart rate over an extended period of time. They are injecting creativity and variety to keep you from getting bored out of your mind and to keep you coming back. But in the end it's still all the same thing - Cardio.

Detach your mind from the work. This is the exact opposite of resistance work where the mind is focused on the exercise. With Cardio let the body operate on its own while the mind is involved with something else to pass the time or step up the motivation.

Don't try to be creative with your Cardio. Don't be looking to make it more interesting. Just the opposite! Keep it as routine and predictable as possible. Tune it out and occupy your time with something else: reading, watching, writing, thinking. Whatever. Just don't focus on it. It's a lot easier when you're not paying attention. Put your time in. Come back tomorrow.

Cardio is a continuation of the same effort while resistance training is a progression of effort.

Twenty minutes for Cardio is a good baseline. You may be able to go longer or you may need to do less. It is important to keep in mind that you only have so much recovery ability to spare. You are adding muscle and losing fat. The body needs to be able to rebuild after the resistance work but it also gets fatigued from the Cardio.

Remember that we always prioritize. Overdoing Cardio will cut into your limited recovery reserves and this will negatively affect muscle gains. Everything must be balanced.

Live and Let Diet

(Eat Right)

Chapter 15

Nutrition

> *Fat, drunk and stupid is no way to go through life son.*
> — Dean Vernon Wormer
> Animal House (1978)

When we talk about nutrition we generally mean the ingestion of what the body needs for good health and growth. The science of nutrition is the study of these effects and how the nutrients relate to the various functions of the body.

Diet then describes the actual content of the food material that is consumed. It doesn't necessarily mean a restriction on the amount of food ingested, but the word has become so associated with weight loss that this is the first thing people think of when they hear the word. Your diet can be actively managed for purposes other than losing weight, such as boosting your overall health or helping to treat some disease conditions.

But diet plans are just information. All the fancy programs and scientific data can't change one simple fact: you have to eat less if you want to reduce fat. All these great plans can't change the one behavior that is needed.

A diet is only as good as the effort put into it to eat less. This is not saying that nutritional content and exercise don't matter, only that the diet itself requires you to take in less calories than you expend.

This is the tough part. Just like an exercise routine. All the commercials that you hear on the radio and see on the TV are merely selling information.

There are too many people out there making this way too complicated purely out of self interest.

Eating

It's really pretty simple: you eat, the food contains calories, your body burns off what it needs and stores the rest away. Too many calories for your level of activity results in accumulating fat. Most diets are based on variations of this to some extent.

An effective plan comes down to two things:

1. Tracking calories
2. Macro-nutrition

Calories are counted because any excess will be stored as fat. The amount of calories must be adjusted according to energy requirements. It's not what you eat. It's what you don't eat that matters.

Macro-nutrition means thinking in terms of protein for tissue building or repair and carbohydrates (carbs) for energy (fuel).

Aim for at least 1/2 gram of protein per pound of body weight. For a 160 pound man consuming 100g of protein per day that means 400 calories from protein, or 20% of the total calories if the maintenance level is 2000 calories per day. This could also be used to calculate projected weight loss. If the calories were limited to 1600/day in this example then this might target a 2 pounds per week weight loss.

A basic nutritional breakdown using this same example could be 20/50/30. That is, 20% of calories from protein, 50% from carbs and 30% from fat.

Food intake must be matched to a less active lifestyle. Time to start thinking about eating more to feed the body and to provide essential nutrients rather than to fuel physical performance.

Your carb intake must align with your lifestyle level of activity. If you sit behind a desk all day you are not living an active lifestyle regardless of how much you exercise.

All calories are not created equal. Carbs should be thought of as fuel and protein as maintenance when meals are considered. Carbs will be burned for energy and excess will be stored as glycogen and then fat. And increasing lean muscle mass usually means consuming a greater portion of your calories from protein.

This may look like a tall order, but with all the fitness apps out there it becomes pretty simple. Many good ones are free and the learning curve is not very steep. Once you get used to doing it, tracking and preparing your food intake becomes easy and routine.

Try out a few of the more popular ones, like MyFitnessPal, until you find one that you like. To get started you enter your weight and activity level (most likely "sedentary" - let's be honest). Next calculate your calorie requirements based on gaining or losing weight. Track your meals and adjust by addressing your protein intake first.

Aim for 20+% protein and keep an eye on the fat percentage as this often fills in quickly with protein rich foods. Finish up by working on the carb component and you will have effectively designed your meal plan according to your specific calorie needs and proper macro-nutrition profile.

Create some base meals and stick with these primarily. Leave the variety for weekends or special occasions. Supplements should take care of vitamin and mineral needs. You cannot be careless about your meals. You can still eat things you enjoy, but they must be planned.

You owe it to yourself to live a little. I don't mean pig out constantly and neglect your diet, but enjoy some buffalo wings and a beer or two now and then. It's not reasonable to be super strict all the time when it comes to eating.

But body fat will blur definition. You cannot naturally carry enough lean muscle to afford a layer of body fat covering up hard earned muscle mass. You need to do your Cardio if you want to look sharp. There is no getting around this.

At some point you may come across the phrase "Eating Clean." It's hard to describe exactly what that means, but it involves limiting meals to whole and unprocessed foods. After that the descriptions go all over the place.

A good visual illustration might be to picture a plain hamburger patty with a baked potato and a side vegetable and compare that to a messy fast food cheeseburger and fries. You get the picture.

Eating clean will yield most of the supposed benefits of organic/healthy/expensive/fussy/preparation-intensive meals. Either way, macros and calories should be your main concern.

Eat Light at Night

The single most effective change to your diet is addressing what you eat before going to bed. Lighten up the evening meal and the pounds will come off. Think higher protein and lower carbs at night.

The toughest part of your diet is what you eat in the evening. If you wake up full and bloated in the morning then you ate too much (or the wrong things) before bed. Digestion was not efficient and you took a step backwards.

You have to eat enough during the day so that you don't come home at night starving. Then you will eat everything in sight and not pay attention to proper nutrition.

This is the game changer. You will not believe the difference this makes in how you look and how you feel. So many people try so hard in the gym and put in the effort to improve their physical state and then just blow it by not paying enough attention to diet.

The simple step of limiting your evening meal will get you most of the way to managing your diet efforts. Your body will respond quickly and dramatically. You won't have a belly full of food that needs to be digested when the body is trying to rest and recover. You won't wake up bloated and sluggish. You sleep well and can better appreciate the effort you put in at the gym. You will see your body leaning out, getting cut, and starting to develop a muscular look.

You will never want to go back to your old evening eating habits.

Supplements

Earlier we mentioned that supplements should take care of vitamin and mineral needs.

Of course, it's a little more involved than that.

A nutritional supplement can be anything added to your dietary intake as long as it is not marketed as a regular food or drug. Laws define what supplements cannot claim to be, but the government does not approve them for sale (although they may determine safety in some cases).

As you might imagine, there are so many varieties of supplements that it's hard to decide where to even start. For our purpose, and the sake of our sanity, we will limit the discussion to the types of supplements that are intended to promote lean body mass. Think of lean body mass as the inverse of body fat percentage.

Protein

When it comes to building muscle the first consideration is supplementing protein intake. Protein synthesis becomes elevated after resistance training and therefore requires greater intake of protein in order to gain lean muscle tissue. Meat, poultry, seafood and eggs all represent high-quality dietary protein, but for lower cost and convenience a readily available protein source is also advantageous.

Protein supplements can be purchased as powders, pre-mixed shakes, bars or other forms intended to be eaten as is or added to a meal or drink, generally after a workout. Powders are the most popular and usually the most cost effective. They come in a wide variety of flavors and can be mixed with water, milk or juice as desired. Protein powder is primarily taken after exercise but many people substitute protein supplements for regular meals or take them at other times for their particular protein intake needs.

Whey protein is very popular and is often thought of as superior to other protein sources for muscle growth following resistance exercise. Whey is produced from milk and is processed in several different forms in an effort to increase effectiveness. You will usually find whey sold as a powder, sometimes in very large containers, which then gets mixed with water or some other beverage for consuming after a workout.

Creatine

Creatine is a supplement that is taken to enhance performance during resistance training exercise. It's rather well thought of in this capacity and has received support from professional organizations in sports medicine and nutrition. It works by providing energy to muscle cells in the course of intense activity that's brief and repetitive, as you would see when lifting weights.

The Drink Cooler

What is all this stuff in the refrigerator?

The bottles of water I can figure out, but everything else? Will the juice, sodas and other sweet drinks help me reach my goals?

Pre-workout

As you might assume, pre-workout supplements are intended to be taken prior to working out and are designed to help get you started and keep you going through your session. These products are meant to help support increased energy, concentration, and stamina in the gym. Different brands include a variety of ingredients with one of the most common being caffeine. If you're already a coffee drinker then you have a good idea of what to expect.

Sports Drinks

Think Gatorade, which has the bulk of the market in the U.S. The idea is to replace the water and electrolytes that you lose when you sweat during exercise. Electrolytes are really just salts. Calcium, sodium and potassium mainly, which the body needs at sufficient levels for adequate muscle contraction and to avoid muscle weakness. These drinks also provide calories from carbs to support exercise performance. Without exercise, consuming too many sports drinks can lead to weight gain just like over consumption of sodas or any other high calorie beverages.

Energy Drinks

Where sports drinks are meant to improve athletic activities, energy drinks are designed to act as a stimulant whether exercising or not. Caffeine is usually present in these drinks, along with a variety of other ingredients intended to improve physical performance and alertness. Energy drinks may also be carbonated and/or sweetened with many different brands offering a wide assortment to choose from. Red Bull is probably the most widely known drink in this group.

Lactose Intolerance

Milk and other dairy products have long been recognized as basic protein sources for *Muscle Building*. Consuming protein soon after proper lifting activity has always been considered an effective means of promoting muscle growth.

Unfortunately many of us will experience difficulty with digesting milk-based protein later in life.

Lactose intolerance occurs when your body does not have enough of the intestinal enzyme lactase to break down the sugar in milk products (lactose).

The symptoms can vary in severity but usually include bloating, diarrhea and abdominal discomfort to some degree. A lot of this depends on how much dairy you have consumed and how much your lactase level has declined over time.

You may only have trouble after multiple glasses of milk or a pint of ice cream, or you may begin to suffer just from adding some half & half to your coffee. Either way some adjustments need to be made.

The point is that you may no longer be able to address your protein requirements with milk and milk-based products. As these sorts of things are very common with younger people looking to put on muscle, many of us in middle age are going to have to find alternatives.

Your fitness app can be a big help in searching out foods to replace the dairy protein that you can no longer tolerate. Remember to track your calories and stay within your macro-nutrition ranges and you should find that you won't miss milk as much as you thought. And of course you'll feel that much better as those distressing symptoms fade away.

Whey Protein

Protein powders are very popular nutritional supplements in the fitness world. These supplements may be derived from any number of protein sources, but it's pretty much agreed that the highest quality comes from whey. When milk is curdled, the liquid whey is strained out and processed into powder form.

Regardless of the benefits, proceed with caution. As a milk derivative, whey contains lactose and may bring on the same symptoms as any other dairy product.

The Rest Will
Take Care of Itself
(Recover, Restore, Replenish)

Chapter 16

Sleep

> *Early to bed and early to rise, makes a man healthy, wealthy, and wise*
> — Benjamin Franklin (1706-1790)
> American statesman, scientist and philosopher

As we mentioned earlier, muscle actually grows when the body is resting, not when you are exercising in the gym. Sleep allows the body to revive and rejuvenate while providing a favorable environment for greater physical development.

When we sleep our bodies enter into an anabolic, or building up state. At the risk of starting a Biochemistry lecture, suffice it to say that as the metabolism slows down, conditions in our muscle cells become favorable for synthesizing additional muscle tissue.

The biochemical reactions that take place during sleep are responsible for the increases in muscle mass. In addition to muscle, the majority of the other body structures enter into an anabolic state during sleep.

Nerves, bones and organs are also all repaired and revitalized at this time. Sleep also allows for the removal of metabolic waste products and is essential for keeping a healthy immune system.

Tips for Better Sleep

If *Muscle Building* really takes place when you're asleep, it stands to reason that putting a little effort into sleeping better would be to your benefit. The quality of your rest directly impacts recovery from your physical exertion. You break it down in the gym and build it back up when you sleep.

There aren't any real secrets here, and most of the advice on improving sleep comes down to a few basic categories and some common sense.

The first tip has been mentioned before:

Eat Light at Night

Not only does this help your fat burning, but not having heavy food sitting in your stomach overnight will make it easier on your digestive system and leave more of your body's resources available to help restore and strengthen your tired muscles.

Also you will want to watch the amount of fluids you drink right before bed. We all tend to dehydrate somewhat overnight so taking in some water is not a bad idea. Too much and you'll be waking up during the night for trips to the bathroom, so it pays to find the ideal amount that just gets you through the night without waking up parched. On a related note, it shouldn't be news to anyone that alcohol or coffee before bed are not going to result in the most restful night's sleep, though for different reasons.

The second tip is pretty obvious but with lots of variables:

Establish the Best Possible Bedroom Conditions

Keep It Cool

Lower the thermostat to around 65, turn on the overhead fan and/or open the window a little to keep the air circulating and the room adequately ventilated. Your body temperature drops as you sleep and a temperature that's too high could interfere with that. If your partner prefers (demands?) a warmer room then try to suggest some flannel pajamas (good luck - but seriously try to work out some kind of compromise because it is important and makes a huge difference).

Get Dark

For most people, the body reacts naturally to darkness. The hormone that regulates sleep, melatonin, is released in response to dark conditions. Unfortunately the level of this hormone decreases with age so it becomes even more important in later years to minimize light when sleeping.

Quiet on the Set

Again, no secret here, but minor noise during the night could interfere with the quality of your sleep even if it's not loud enough to wake you up. Shut the door, turn off the TV, close the window and turn up the A/C if there is anything outside disturbing you. Maybe try out some "white noise" to drown out anything that may be bothering you. Look for free phone apps if this interests you before investing in a stand-alone machine that may not be necessary.

And a couple more tips:

Stay on Schedule

Tuning in to your body's natural cycle of falling asleep and waking up will help to maximize your sleep quality and physical restoration. We all have various biological rhythms that influence or control daily repeating processes such as eating and sleeping. Going to sleep and getting out of bed at consistent times will keep the internal clock on track and benefit your overall rest and recovery. If you find yourself needing more sleep than you're getting at night it's alright to make it up with naps, just try not to disrupt the natural cycle too much. Or if you sleep in late on the weekend don't adjust by staying up much later than usual. In other words get back on schedule as soon as you can.

Relax and Unwind

Get into a routine each night where you go through some basic preparations for the next day where you're not stressing out or causing yourself to worry over something. Watch (a little) TV, take a shower, get your next day's clothes together, read a book, set the alarm, anything that is simple and calming that you can do without thinking about it too much. Try to do the same things every night and your body will begin to recognize this as a sign to call it a day.

You Look Mahvelous
(Appearance Counts)

Chapter 17

Appearance

> *Dahling, I have to tell you something.*
> *And I don't say this to everybody.*
> *You look mahvelous!*
>
> — Billy Crystal, Fernando's Hideaway,
> Saturday Night Live (1985)

And now we come to, maybe for some, the most important topic - looking better.

Like it or not, details of your physical attributes may be thought of as more or less appealing by others. Some of these features are common everywhere and some are relative, both at the individual and at the group cultural level.

There is obviously unlimited variation in physical appearance with many factors being genetic and many others coming from active effort on your part. Basic size and coloration is pretty much determined by nature and most people experience long-term physiological changes as they age, generally not for the better.

Clothes, hairstyles and cosmetics are some of the things that people will make use of to vary and improve their appearance. However, it's a lot tougher to change your general body shape as this is mostly determined by skeletal proportions and the particular degree of musculature and fat. Even though genetics are the main determinant, muscle mass can certainly be augmented and reshaped while fat distribution can be altered with proper attention. In addition, your weight can influence posture and how you walk which further impacts the perception of your body's shape.

Further complicating the dynamics of appearance is the concept of body image, or your own impression of the attractiveness of your body. Your appreciation of your own physical characteristics may not be in tune with whatever ideals you believe others look for. This can come from a blend of expectations, comparisons and perceptions of various standards and often leads to an impulse to lose weight when feeling less positive about what you see in the mirror.

Look Better

A little muscle and a lot less fat goes a long way. Usually the first body part to show results is the arms. Why do you think this is? Because there's very little fat on the arms, at least relative to the abdomen, hips, etc. It's not just about getting bigger. Don't mistake bulk for building muscle. Bulk is a little bit of muscle covered by a lot more body fat. Once the pecs start to swell a little and the shirtsleeves get tighter it's easy to fall into the bulking trap. Lifting heavier, resting more, blowing off Cardio. All of this is counterproductive to the goal of increasing lean body mass. You can't flex fat.

By applying the principles of *Muscle Building* and following the recommended strategy for Cardio and diet, you will enhance your physical attractiveness by approaching social and cultural ideals of body shape. Follow this up with clothing that displays your new traits and add some age appropriate grooming techniques and you will be showing the world a healthier and more youthful body.

For men, a suit with a tailored cut shows off the build. Slim or fitted hugs the body more. You may need to start buying suit separates if your chest measurement is more than 8-10 inches over your waist. With a bigger suit jacket you'll probably need alterations to take in the lower part. Don't be afraid to show a little cuff by taking up the sleeve length.

Skin just looks better with a tan. There are many ways to go here, from natural to all kinds of products. You may just like a new look.

The Best is Yet to Come
(Inspiration)

Chapter 18

Believe

> *Most men lead lives of quiet desperation ...*
> *(notably quoted in the 1987 film Dead Poets Society)*
> — Henry David Thoreau (1817-1862) American poet

It is said that youth is wasted on the young.

Reclaim your youth while keeping the insight and perspective that comes with experience.

Look forward to your next birthday knowing that you will be better physically and your growth will continue for years to come.

The way to get started is to stop thinking about it. Just get yourself to the gym and start. You get going by warming up and stretching, easy stuff that you can do with very little effort. The point is to build some momentum and prepare yourself for the harder work that will follow. This is easier on you mentally than forced discipline (which can be very tough to keep up over a longer period of time).

Commit

Commit to an hour a day, five days a week.

All things are possible if you make time for them.

If you ever were in really good shape when you were younger you will be quite pleased with your results. You never expected that you could look this way again.

If you've never been particularly fit or athletic at any point in your life you will be astonished. If you couldn't get into this kind of shape in your youth how is it possible to look and feel this good at this age?

There really is no excuse.

Everyone gets the same 24 hours per day.

Discipline is contagious.

The more you force yourself to do something the easier and more routine it becomes.

You won't struggle to get yourself to do it.

You miss it if you don't do it.

Progress Not Perfection

Our mission is to show the legions of desperate, middle aged desk jockeys that there is a better way - you don't have to fall apart, it's not inevitable.

Rocky coached Adonis (Apollo Creed's son if you didn't see the movie): one step at a time, one punch at a time, one round at a time.

We can apply that same guidance to our training:

One rep at a time
One set at a time
One body part at a time

Basically this means focus on what you're doing. Don't be looking ahead and worrying about what's to come.

Positive thoughts in the moment always improves the experience. Develop an awareness of this and catch yourself when you start thinking negative thoughts. Think of something positive and watch how fast it turns around. I especially notice this when doing Cardio. Cardio works best when you can detach from the activity and let the body perform automatically. I notice when the negative thoughts creep in that the performance starts to drag. The resistance feels harder and I'm just trying to finish up and get off the machine. When I'm able to turn my thoughts around and embrace something more pleasant or something that

I'm looking forward to then it gets to be fun again. I sail through the motion and I'm even disappointed when it's time to stop.

Chapter 19

Achieve

> *The starting point of all achievement is desire.*
> *Keep this constantly in mind.*
> — Napoleon Hill (1883-1970)
> American motivational writer

Finally, it's here.

The plan for everyone who made it through adolescence, survived high school, turned into a weekend warrior as a young adult and wondered if anyone was going to come up with something that really worked for all those later years.

Don't be fooled by programs that promise results by making you leaner, stronger or give you more stamina.

The most important thing for middle age is mass. Adding more muscle should be your first priority. Cutting excess fat and improving your cardio/respiratory health come next but the quality of your life as you age is directly impacted by the muscle you keep. The wasting away of your body can only be arrested by building your body. Whether you want this for appearance, health or longevity is up to you but first you need to get your approach straight.

Everyone thinks you have to turn up the intensity to the point of passing out. Or push yourself constantly to do something more than before. No wonder so many burn out or get frustrated with the lack of results for all your efforts.

None of this is necessary or even productive. Your exercise routine should be challenging in a reasonable way and repeatable so that you are not constantly living in fear of failing to accomplish what you've been tasked with.

Simply do the work the right way, day in and day out, week after week and watch the results come in.

Muscle mass is not the same as muscle strength. There is a fundamental distinction between these two concepts that makes all the difference in the world. This changes the approach to training and requires a completely new mindset and execution.

Gone is lifting to failure and taking ridiculous amounts of time to rest before attempting the next lift to fail at. You simply stay in the 10 - 12 rep range where the set becomes challenging to finish but you always stop short of failure. It is critical to save something for the next set. In other words you always leave a little left in the tank. Maybe at the end of the workout you can go all out, but the goal is always to get the reps in. This is the protocol that must be followed to increase muscle tissue and reverse the loss of lean body mass that naturally accompanies age once you reach midlife.

Everything is Better When You're Good at It

Stay ahead of the deterioration curve!

There are hundreds of tweaks and adjustments that increase efficiency and results without requiring any more time or effort.

Build your body!

Stop worrying about how many reps you can do or how fast you can run. Who cares if you rode your bike 100 miles this weekend or you went jogging three days in a row. Your body is going to wear down over time and your efforts need to go towards reversing that trend.

Unfortunately at a certain point neglect and deterioration can lead to injuries and/or physical conditions that you may not be able to come back from. Taking charge sooner rather than later is the best response to prevent this from happening. How many people do you know that have had surgery that severely limits their activity? Or medical events, e.g. heart attack, that changes their life irreparably? You need to challenge your body every week so that it must respond by strengthening and repairing itself. Lean muscle tissue will build itself up so you don't waste away. Your pulmonary system and cardio processes should be continually regenerating, heart and lungs getting stronger and more efficient.

Chapter 20

Expect

> *Many of life's failures are people who did not realize how close they were to success when they gave up.*
> — Thomas Alva Edison (1847-1931)
> American inventor

Don't be fooled by all the "life is short" stuff out there. We are here a long time and you don't want to spend half or more of your time here as a decrepit, broken down wreck just hanging on instead of enjoying yourself and living life to the fullest.

Remember that first Spiderman movie? Peter Parker gets bitten by a radioactive spider during a school field trip to some research lab. He wakes up the next morning to a new muscular physique which he checks out in the mirror approvingly. Then he puts on his glasses only to discover that his eyesight has improved and he doesn't need the specs anymore.

That's a pretty good description of how you will feel when you get your physical attributes to start growing again (well without the wall crawling and web swinging). Visible, noticeable, functional improvements that will change your outlook on life and inspire you to continue what you're doing because you know you will keep getting better as time goes on.

If you don't want to look like an old man or woman there are some things to pay attention to right away.

The first thing that gives you away is the breakdown in the shoulder girdle. Scrawny, weak and hunched over is no way to go through life. The shoulders, upper chest and traps should be prioritized if you're really in bad shape.

I see plenty of mid-lifers in the gym working their arms and sitting back on the recumbent bike trying to drop a few pounds. And you will probably see quick results in your biceps because there usually isn't much fat there and you use your arms every day. Of course they will respond and give you that visual feedback that keeps you coming back. Same thing with the easy Cardio. It's not so hard to do and before you know it your pants are a little looser in the waist.

Wow, you're on your way! Can't wait to get to the gym tomorrow.

But beyond that you still look your age (or worse). Sunken chest, slouched posture, toothpick legs. Your approach needs to align with this stage of your life and the goals that you should be working towards: look younger, feel better, live longer. Built to Last.

The joy comes from knowing that you are on the right path and that your efforts are worth it. You can look forward to the years ahead with the confidence that you will be better than you are today.

I'm not talking about losing a few pounds or curling a 25 pound dumbbell instead of a 15. This is about adding lean muscle mass at a time when your body naturally tends to lose muscle and accelerates the aging process. What we're doing is reversing this trend and putting you on the path to recapture your youth and vitality.

It's the midlife miracle.

Not the Biggest, Strongest or Most Aerobic

But very advanced in all three areas.

If you want to stay young you need to build muscle. Not get "toned"so you can squeeze into your new Slim Fit suit. If you want to reverse aging you need to up your muscle mass.

This doesn't just happen randomly because you decided to drag yourself into the gym and listen to some 22 year old who only cares about taking selfies and putting them up on Instagram to get a million followers.

The original Pumping Iron had a song that said it best: Do you want to live forever. Not sure if they were talking about everlasting fame (I doubt it) but more like taking control of your health by building your body instead of letting it deteriorate over time like most everyone else.

You should be doing everything exactly right and appropriate for how you live at this point in your life. You can't just listen to what some other fitness enthusiast is telling you to do or try to recapture the glory of your high school athletics days. It won't work for you at this stage of your life, or at least you won't be getting the results you should be getting. Instead you'll probably experience a lot of frustration and possibly a few new injuries for all your efforts.

I read an article in the newspaper about a Ninja Warrior on some TV show and her training and nutrition methods. She says that she never thinks about exercise as keeping in shape. She thinks about the skills that she needs (I guess to be a Ninja) and which muscles need to be developed to perform those skills.

This is the polar opposite of what we are talking about in Built to Last. The last thing you should be concerned with during your training is how this is going to help you do something else. If you want to work on your golf swing or become a Ninja or anything else then train for that. We are concerned with exercise and nutrition that slows or reverses the natural loss of muscle as you age. This is the end goal for all your efforts. If it also makes you a better Ninja then it's a bonus.

I Can't Wait Until I Reach 60

It occurred to me as I was thinking about my next birthday, that I see no reason to be in any lesser (if not better) shape than I'm in now. I feel no different than at 50 and think I look even better now. I have refined my approach and employ a workable routine that allows me to improve my physical self continually.

I asked for some new workout clothes for Father's Day. When I opened up the presents my wife looked at the new clothes as I held them up and said they were huge, too big. I got all XX sizes which I wear a lot but they still look big when new. First time wearing them in the gym and guess what - they just fit. Not baggy, not even loose, just fit right. I have reached the holy grail of fitness - I got bigger while my weight didn't go up, actually went down. The program works.

My young son just paid me the highest compliment. I was pumping up an inflatable pool toy for him and he was watching me fill it up with the bicycle pump in my bathing suit. All of a sudden he says "Dad, you're really ripped." Wanting to be sure I knew what he meant I asked him what he was talking about. He said "you know ..." and did a sort of muscle pose. Then he said all his friends say the same thing about me.

How many adults do you know who's feet keep growing? In the last 15-20 years my shoe size has gone from a size 9 to a size 10 1/2. I'm not saying my foot is getting longer but it is getting bigger. Like all my other body parts my feet are growing because the muscles are getting bigger and thicker. Plenty of middle age guys need bigger clothes (and especially bigger pants) as they get older but it has nothing to do with an increase in muscle size. I remember back in my early 20's (when presumably you are finished growing) being a size 8 or 8 1/2 so wearing a 10 1/2 at this stage of my life is remarkable.

Chapter 21

Observe

> *If we did all the things we are capable of doing, we would literally astonish ourselves.*
>
> — Thomas Alva Edison (1847-1931)
> American inventor

There's always this fear, this anxiety, that your health is slipping away or that there's nothing you can do about it.

Take charge of your health and your life. Don't wait for something to go wrong or just gradually break down. You can renew yourself and revitalize your physical being.

So many people come into the gym after being away for a long time and start working out from where they left off in High School.

Stop it already. You're not a teenager and you're not a professional athlete. You're not in here to train for performance. Your priorities are different now. This is for Life. You can spot the ones who used to play organized sports when younger. They're probably looking back to those days thinking "I can still do that".

It takes a whole different approach now. Same tools, different reasons.

You are here to build your body: add muscle, lose fat, develop better heart and lungs, more efficient metabolism, and the appearance and outlook of someone who's got all that.

Sometimes older people in the gym can look somewhat impressive from a distance. As you get closer you notice the look comes from exposed toned arms and dressing like a gym rat. Throw in a little attitude and it seems like you got something going. But up close you see the scrawniness and lack of overall vitality. What's missing is the muscle mass.

Occasionally you will come across someone in middle age who really looks great, bragging about their awesome fitness routine and healthy lifestyle. Inevitably it will come out that they have some unusual set of circumstances that allows them a good deal of free time that they happily devote to hanging around the gym all day or pursuing other athletic outlets at their leisure. This is not a realistic model for the vast majority of mid-lifers whose schedules are tight and whose obligations to others, spouse, kids, etc. are the priority. Much as we'd all love to devote all our time to our own personal enjoyment and betterment, it's just not going to happen anytime soon.

You see plenty of kids walking around in tank tops - cut to the max, v-taper, vascular. A little muscle pump on a skinny body can look impressive to the untrained eye.

That not what we are after here.

You may be getting stronger, leaning out, toning up.

But you're not building muscle.

You're not increasing your lean muscle mass.

And if you're not doing that in middle age then you're deteriorating physically. You need to be adding muscle just to counter the natural effects of aging. Never mind actually growing and adding additional muscle. Doing this requires a specific dedicated approach.

You're Doing Yourself a Favor

You are doing yourself an enormous favor when you know exactly what you're going to do before you get to the gym.

No picking and choosing or wandering around. No anxiety over whether you should be doing this or that.

When you have your workout planned to the letter you move through it with more authority. No self doubt or distractions over what anyone else is doing. Get in, get out. Do a good job and come back tomorrow and do it better. Solid, steady improvement will be yours.

The human body is capable of performing almost an unlimited variety of movements and motions. There really is no end to the number of variations that your muscles can do.

If you find yourself doing something that feels odd or looks weird, or if someone is showing you some variation that you never saw before ask yourself what this is trying to accomplish. What is the goal of doing it this way?

Recap

Chapter 22

Taking Care of Business

> *You cannot escape the responsibility of tomorrow by evading it today*
> — Abraham Lincoln (1809-1865)
> 16th President of the United States

The workouts are sustainable, and the gains continue to progress because you're not pushing yourself to the limit every time.

The amount of work you do is what triggers the response.

You don't burn out and you don't get bored because there is an endless variety of tweaks and improvements that you can do. Experiment and test your enhancements.

The biggest mistake I see people make is lifting for strength.

Increasing strength is a critical component but it is not the primary goal. Our program uses strength, but the exercise methods are not focused on this.

Muscle Building requires a different approach.

Stop worrying about how much weight you're using. Stick with the weight that gets you 10-12 reps per set for all the sets you're doing.

Here's a classic example: you do 185 on the bench for 10 reps. Next week you only get 185 for 8. Oh no! I'm going backwards, it's not working. You skip your next workout out of disgust. Before you know it you're not going to the gym at all.

You can't imagine what a relief it is to not worry about how much you're lifting. No performance anxiety. When it's time to move the weight up your body will feel it and you'll know it intuitively.

The second biggest mistake is exercising just to lose weight. Of course, reducing fat is important, but just like lifting for strength it is not the primary goal. Cardio should be as mindless as possible. Music, TV, movie, reading or some combination of these. Just put the time in at the right resistance level and don't think about it anymore.

A recent trend with men is to blame a declining physical condition on a low level of testosterone. Whether there is some condition causing it or whether it's the natural consequence of aging, there seems to be no shortage of solutions to get the body producing more testosterone or to introduce it externally.

My response is simple: why would the body produce more testosterone if it doesn't need it? If you live a sedentary lifestyle and make no effort to counter the natural effects of aging (meaning the continual loss of muscle) then you should expect lower levels of this hormone.

Adding testosterone and then expecting the body to respond with growth when it has no reason to makes no sense. When the body is stimulated properly to add muscle then it will produce more testosterone, not the opposite.

The best way to counter aging is to discourage your body from getting old. Medicine, pharmaceuticals, nutritional supplementation, genetic manipulation and any related tech all address the issue after the fact.

The answer is to not let yourself deteriorate in the first place, or at least slow it down to avoid most of the detrimental effects of aging.

Chapter 23

Never Give Up

> *Our greatest weakness lies in giving up.*
> *The most certain way to succeed is*
> *always to try just one more time.*
>
> — Thomas Alva Edison (1847-1931)
> American inventor

So many people try it for a while and don't get the results they're looking for.

Why put in the effort if you're not getting anything out of it?

This works. You can keep on going with the confidence and reassurance that comes with knowing you're on the right track.

If you need variety to motivate you then you're in the wrong place. We are after a lot more than simply exercising because we know we should and just worrying about getting bored.

Your goal is to get to the point where your efforts are almost machine-like. Same workouts week after week.

This is the formula - deviate at your own risk. There's plenty of room for personal preference and individual variation as you execute the movements and choose your Cardio. But the framework stays in place.

Chapter 24

Final Thoughts

> *And in the end, it's not the years in your life that count. It's the life in your years.*
>
> — Abraham Lincoln (1809-1865)
> 16th President of the United States

So, in summary, you don't have to kill yourself with exercise - you just need to do the work.

You don't have to push yourself to the point of exhaustion or try for a new personal best every time. But you do need to put the time in and complete enough volume of repetition to trigger the muscles of the body to grow.

A sound fundamental approach is all that's required. Good form, a reasonably challenging level of resistance, proper management of rest time along with basic attention to nutrition and respect for the importance of recuperation and you'll be on your way.

Years of neglect will eventually catch up with you. Like anything else that needs to work properly, without regular maintenance and upkeep sooner or later it will break down.

But not if you are Built to Last!

Acknowledgements

I would like to thank my amazing wife Maura, and my wonderful children, Kayla and Nick. Your love and support are always present and your unending belief in me makes all things possible and all my efforts worth it.

Made in the USA
Middletown, DE
24 June 2021